POTS SYNDROME COOKBOOK: FOR BEGINNERS AND NEWLY DIAGNOSED

A Quick and Easy Guide to Managing Postural Orthostatic Tachycardia Syndrome, Improving Blood Volume and Circulation

Dr. Anna Fennell

COPYRIGHT

Copyright © 2024 by Dr. Anna Fennell

TABLE OF CONTENTS

DELICIOUS POTS SYNDROME DIET DINNER RECIPES

CHAPTER ONE

OVERVIEW OF POTS SYNDROME

Postural orthostatic tachycardia syndrome (POTS) is a condition that causes your heart to beat faster than normal when you transition from sitting or lying down to standing up. It's a type of orthostatic intolerance.

Each word of "postural orthostatic tachycardia syndrome" has a meaning:

Postural: Related to the position of your body.

Orthostatic: Related to standing upright.

Tachycardia: A heart rate over 100 beats per minute.

Syndrome: A group of symptoms that happen together.

Normally, your body's autonomic nervous system balances your heart rate and blood pressure to keep your blood flowing at a healthy pace, no matter what position your body is in. If you have POTS, your body can't coordinate the balancing act of blood vessel constriction (squeezing) and heart rate response. This means that your body can't keep your blood pressure steady and stable. This causes a variety of symptoms.

Each case of POTS is different. People with POTS may see symptoms come and go over a period of years. In most cases, with adjustments in diet, medications and physical activity, a person with POTS will experience an improvement in their quality of life.

Who does POTS affect?

The majority of people with POTS are women and people assigned female at birth aged 15 to 50 years.

But men and people assigned male at birth can also have POTS.

You're at a higher risk of developing POTS after experiencing the following stressors:

Significant illnesses, such as viral illnesses like mononucleosis or serious infections.

Pregnancy.

Physical trauma, such as a head injury.

Surgery.

People who have certain autoimmune conditions, such as Sjogren's syndrome, lupus and celiac disease, are also more likely to develop POTS.

How common is POTS?

POTS is common. It affects about 1 to 3 million people in the United States.

Types and Causes of POTS

The causes of POTS vary from person to person. Researchers don't entirely understand the origins of this disorder. The classification of POTS is the subject of discussion, but most authorities recognize different characteristics in POTS, which occur in some patients more than others. Importantly, these characteristics are not mutually exclusive; person with POTS may experience more than of these at the same time:

Neuropathic POTS is a term used to describe POTS associated with damage to the small fiber nerves (small-fiber neuropathy). These nerves regulate the constriction of the blood vessels in the limbs and abdomen.

Hyperadrenergic POTS is a term used to describe POTS associated with elevated levels of the stress hormone norepinephrine.

Hypovolemic POTS is a term used to describe POTS associated with abnormally low levels of blood (hypovolemia).

Secondary POTS means that POTS is associated with another condition known to potentially cause autonomic neuropathy, such as diabetes, Lyme disease, or autoimmune disorders such as lupus or Sjögren's syndrome.

POTS Risk Factors

Dysautonomia International estimates that POTS affects between one and three million people in the U.S. The majority of them are women, although men may also develop POTS. POTS is less common in young children, but it affects adolescents, and symptoms often develop during puberty. POTS may begin after an apparent or confirmed viral illness, but it can also appear following surgery and other health events.

POTS can run in families, but no single gene associated with the majority of cases of POTS has been identified. A mutation in the norepinephrine transporter gene appears to affect only a tiny portion of POTS patients. Among genetic factors, there is a strong association between POTS and various joint hypermobility disorders, including Ehlers-Danlos syndrome. Recent research has also highlighted an overlap between POTS, joint hypermobility and mast cell disorders, some of which have a genetic origin.

Common Symptoms and Manifestations

What are the symptoms of postural orthostatic tachycardia syndrome?

POTS symptoms vary from person to person and may include:

Severe and/or long-lasting fatigue

Lightheadedness with prolonged sitting or standing that can lead to fainting

Brain fog: trouble focusing, remembering or paying attention

Forceful heartbeats or heart palpitations (a feeling of the heart pounding or skipping a beat)

Nausea and vomiting

Headaches

Excessive sweating

Shakiness

Intolerance of exercise or a prolonged worsening of general symptoms after increased activity

A pale face and purple discoloration of the hands and feet if the limbs are lower than the level of the heart

POTS symptoms typically get worse:

In warm environments, such as a hot bath or shower, a hot room or on a hot day

In situations involving a lot of standing, such as waiting for a bus or when shopping

If fluid and salt intake have not been adequate, such as after skipping a meal

eating, especially refined carbohydrates like white bread

not drinking enough fluids

drinking alcohol

resting too much

exercise

being on your period

POTS symptoms may also get worse when you get a common cold or an infection. In severe cases, POTS symptoms can prevent a person from being upright for more than a couple of minutes. This can greatly affect all aspects of personal, school, work and social life.

Although the origin of POTS symptoms is physical, sometimes people attribute the symptoms incorrectly to psychological disorders such as anxiety. While some people with POTS have anxiety disorders similar to the general population, POTS is not caused by anxiety.

Diagnosis

How is postural orthostatic tachycardia syndrome (POTS) diagnosed?

POTS can be difficult for healthcare providers to diagnose due to the many symptoms that can occur over time. People with POTS may have symptoms for months to years before finally being diagnosed with the condition.

A healthcare provider will ask questions about your symptoms, medications and medical history. They'll also perform a physical exam.

A tilt table test is the main way providers diagnose POTS. During the tilt table test, you are secured on a table while lying flat. Then the table is raised to an almost upright position. Your heart rate, blood pressure and often blood oxygen and exhaled carbon dioxide levels are measured during this test.

You might have POTS if you meet all three of these criteria:

Your body produces an abnormal heart rate response to being upright

Your symptoms worsen when upright

You don't develop orthostatic hypotension in the first three minutes of testing

Besides the tilt table test, your provider may order other tests to help confirm a POTS diagnosis or rule out other possible causes of your symptoms, including:

Blood and urine tests for causes of POTS and conditions that mimic POTS.

QSART (a test that measures the autonomic nerves that control sweating).

Autonomic breathing test (this measures your blood rate and pressure response during exercise).

TST (tuberculin skin test).

Skin nerve biopsy.

Echocardiogram.

Blood volume with hemodynamic studies.

Treatment strategies

Management and Treatment

What is the treatment for postural orthostatic tachycardia syndrome (POTS)?

Unfortunately, there's no cure for POTS. Instead, healthcare providers use several strategies to manage the symptoms of POTS. Treatment is highly individualized based on your symptoms and what works best for you.

The main forms of treatment include:

Exercise and physical activity.

Diet and nutrition.

Medical compression stockings can also help push blood up from your legs to reduce POTS symptoms.

Exercise and physical activity

Exercise and physical activity are key to managing POTS.

Although most people with POTS have healthy hearts, your provider may recommend a cardiac rehab program. This exercise template uses the cardiac rehab model to recondition and help improve health and manage POTS. Some of the best data for treating POTS comes from cardiac rehab.

Studies show that reclined aerobic exercise, such as swimming, rowing and recumbent bicycling, has the best results. Strengthening your core and leg muscles is also helpful.

Here are important things to know as you undergo an exercise program and other physical activities. Talk with your provider for specific instructions on these exercises.

Practice isometric exercises: These exercises involve contracting your muscles without actually moving your body. Isometrics squeeze your muscle and push your blood back toward your heart. They're simple to do, and you can do them lying in bed or seated. It's a good idea to do these in bed before getting up to prepare your body for sitting and standing.

Transition slowly with your body: Go from lying to sitting on the edge of your bed. Stay there for several minutes, allowing your body to naturally adjust to the change in position. Once you're standing, pause and wait before walking to allow your blood pressure to adjust again. If you feel lightheaded at any point, wait for a few minutes in that position to see if it resolves. If not, then return to the prior position. Moving slowly is the key.

Begin a modest walking program: Count how many steps you can do without causing symptoms. These steps are your initial baseline. Start with walking once a day and go a little farther in time, distance or by adding steps. If you feel good, add a second walk in the day. A simple strategy for counting steps is to do 100 to 300 steps per hour during the day. Fitness trackers can monitor steps easily. Every week or every few weeks, add more steps to your daily total.

Practice simple yoga: Practicing basic yoga with a focus on breathing may help reduce POTS symptoms.

CHAPTER TWO

POTS SYNDROME AND DIET

Managing diet and nutrition is another important aspect of managing POTS symptoms.

If you have the hypovolemic (low blood volume) form of POTS, your healthcare provider will likely recommend increasing both your fluid and salt intake to increase blood volume.

Eating a large meal can make symptoms of POTS worse, as your body redirects a lot of blood to aid in the digestion process. Because of this, providers often recommend eating several smaller meals throughout the day instead of two or three large ones.

A nutritionist or dietitian can help you with your diet. This consult can be especially helpful if you have celiac disease or other dietary sensitivities.

General Dietary Guidelines

General guidelines for dietary changes include:

Increase sodium in your diet from 3,000 milligrams (mg) to 10,000 mg per day.

Drink 2 to 2.5 liters per day of fluids. Water is the best choice.

Eat small and frequent meals instead of a few large meals.

Eating a diet with high fiber and complex carbohydrates may help reduce blood glucose (sugar) spikes and lessen POTS symptoms.

Keep your nutrition balanced with protein, vegetables, dairy and fruits.

Choose beneficial salty snacks such as broth, pickles, olives, sardines, anchovies and nuts. Don't over-rely on snack chips and crackers for salt.

Recommended Foods for POTS Patients

For those grappling with Postural Orthostatic Tachycardia Syndrome (POTS), dietary strategies often revolve around steadying blood sugar levels, ensuring ample hydration, and tackling symptoms like dizziness and fatigue head-on. Here's a rundown of suggested foods:

Hydration: Keeping fluid levels in check is paramount for managing POTS symptoms. While water reigns supreme, electrolyte-packed options such as coconut water or sugar-conscious sports drinks can lend a hand.

Salt: Upping your salt intake can work wonders in bolstering blood volume and easing woes like lightheadedness. Opt for wholesome salt sources like sea salt or Himalayan salt.

Complex Carbohydrates: Slow-releasing energy foods are champions in maintaining stable blood sugar levels. Think along the lines of whole grains like quinoa, brown rice, and oats.

Lean Proteins: Protein steps up to the plate in preserving muscle mass and steadying blood sugar levels. Look to lean protein sources such as chicken, turkey, fish, tofu, and legumes.

Fruits and Vegetables: A colorful array of fruits and veggies delivers essential nutrients, vitamins, minerals, and antioxidants. Diversify your plate with a vibrant mix to ensure a well-rounded nutrient intake.

Trigger Foods and Substances to Limit or Avoid

Some individuals find that certain foods or beverages exacerbate their symptoms. Common triggers include caffeine, alcohol, and heavily processed or sugary foods. Keeping a food diary can also be useful to detect and help identify personal triggers.

Importance of Sodium and Fluid Intake

The foundation of treating POTS is to drink fluids frequently throughout the day. For most POTS patients, the goal is at least 64-80 ounces (about 2-2.5 liters) a day. You would also need to increase your intake of salty foods and add more salt to your diet with a saltshaker or salt tablets. These dietary modifications help keep water in the bloodstream, which helps more blood reach the heart and the brain.

CHAPTER THREE

DELICIOUS RECIPES IDEAS FOR THE POTS SYNDROME

DELICIOUS POTS SYNDROME DIET BREAKFAST RECIPES

Smoked haddock & hollandaise bake with dill & caper fried potatoes

Ingredients

150g baby spinach

2 x 140g undyed smoked haddock fillets

For the cheat's hollandaise

2 egg yolks

1 tsp cornflour

100ml double cream, plus a splash

2 tsp white wine vinegar

For the fried potatoes

500g floury potatoes, peeled and chopped into 3cm chunks

knob of butter

1 tbsp rapeseed oil, plus a drizzle

2 shallots, halved and thinly sliced

1 tbsp capers, drained

small handful dill, leaves picked

1 lemon, zested, then cut into wedges to serve

Preparation

STEP 1

Put the potatoes in a pan and cover with cold water. Bring to the boil, cover with a lid and cook for 7-8 mins until a knife easily pierces them but they still hold their shape. Drain and leave to steam dry. Meanwhile, heat the butter and oil in a frying pan, and when the butter is sizzling, add the shallots. Fry until soft, about 5 mins, then add the potatoes and fry for about 15 mins until crispy on all sides.

STEP 2

While the potatoes are cooking, make the hollandaise. Whisk the yolks and cornflour together until smooth. Add the cream and vinegar, and season well. Pour into a small pan, heat very gently, whisking constantly, until the consistency of custard. If the sauce looks like it's splitting, curdling, or getting too hot, add a splash more cream and whisk vigorously – it should become smooth again. Check the seasoning, adding a little more salt or vinegar if it needs it.

STEP 3

Heat the grill to medium-high. Heat a drizzle more oil in another small, ovenproof frying pan. Add the spinach, season and cook until just wilted. Spread the spinach across the pan and place the haddock fillets on top. Spoon over the hollandaise to cover each fillet. Grill for 10 mins until the fish is flaking and the sauce is browning in patches.

STEP 4

Scatter the potatoes with the capers, dill and lemon zest. Serve alongside the fish with lemon wedges for squeezing over.

Ackee & saltfish

Ingredients

600g boneless salted cod

2 tbsp vegetable oil

1 medium onion, finely chopped

4 garlic cloves, finely chopped

3 spring onions, thinly sliced

1 scotch bonnet pepper, deseeded and finely chopped

1 tsp dried thyme

1 tsp ground pimento (allspice)

½ red pepper, deseeded and finely chopped

½ green pepper, deseeded and finely chopped

1 large tomato, chopped

2 x 540g cans ackee, drained

Preparation

STEP 1

Put the salt cold in your pot and cover with cold water. Bring to the boil, then boil for 5 minutes, drain and add fresh cold water to cover.

STEP 2

Repeat this process until you're happy with the saltiness when tasted; we recommend to boil the fish three times in total for a perfect balance of salt in the fish. Drain and leave to cool. Use a fork to shred the salted cod into pieces and set aside.

STEP 3

Now you'll need a large frying pan. Pour the vegetable oil into the frying pan and place over a high heat. Once the oil is sizzling hot, turn the heat down to low-medium. Add the onion, garlic, spring onions and scotch bonnet, then cook until soft, for around 5-7 minutes.

STEP 4

Add the salted cod, dash in some black pepper, thyme and pimento, then mix it together and cook down for around 3 minutes.

STEP 5

Next, add in the red and green bell peppers, along with your tomato. Mix together and cook down for 2-3 minutes. These Ingredients help to bring a heat balance, so it's not too spicy.

STEP 6

Now you'll need to add in your ackee and dash in a little more black pepper. Fold in the ackee; the ackee is soft so it's important to fold it in very gently – nobody likes mushy ackee.

STEP 7

Once folded in, simmer for 3-5 minutes before serving.

Flatbreads with brunch-style eggs

Ingredients

110g self-raising flour, plus extra for dusting

110g atta or plain wholemeal flour

3 tbsp rapeseed oil, plus extra for the bowl and frying

small knob of butter, melted

For the eggs

1 tbsp olive oil

12 cherry tomatoes, halved

4 large eggs

25g grated cheddar

2 tbsp double cream

Preparation

STEP 1

Sift the flours and 1 tsp salt into a large bowl. Add 1 tbsp of the oil and 150ml warm water. Bring together into a soft but not too sticky dough (you may need up to 175ml water). If it feels too wet, add some flour. If it's too dry, add water.

STEP 2

Tip onto a floured surface and knead for 4-5 mins, or until smooth. Put the dough in an oiled bowl, cover and leave for 30 mins.

STEP 3

Tip onto a floured surface. Divide into six balls and roll each out into a thin, 18-20cm wide circle using a rolling pin. If you prefer, you can divide again into twelve balls to make smaller flatbreads.

STEP 4

Brush a heavy-based pan with oil and cook one flatbread over a high heat for 1-2 mins on each side, or until golden and starting to puff. Put on a plate and brush with butter. Repeat with the rest of the dough.

STEP 5

Meanwhile, for the eggs, heat the oil in a small non-stick pan and cook the tomatoes briefly until just softened. Season. Crack the eggs into the pan, add the cheese and cream, cover and cook for 2 mins. Remove the lid. Cook until the egg whites are set, then serve from the pan with the flatbreads, making sure the pan has cooled a little first.

Winter breakfast hash

Ingredients

375g potatoes, cut into small chunks

1 tbsp rapeseed oil

1 onion (about 200g), chopped

½ tsp caraway seeds

2 garlic cloves, chopped

1 green pepper, deseeded and diced

200g large brussels sprouts, trimmed and sliced

2 eggs

Preparation

STEP 1

Boil the potatoes for 15 mins until tender. Meanwhile, heat the oil in a large non-stick frying pan over a medium heat and fry the onion for 8 mins, stirring frequently until it starts to colour. Add the caraway, garlic, pepper and sprouts and cook for 5 mins more with the lid on the pan so they steam at the same time.

STEP 2

Drain and lightly crush the cooked potatoes using a masher. Stir them into the vegetables and cook for 5-10 mins, turning occasionally so the mixture browns.

STEP 3

Meanwhile, poach the eggs for a few minutes for a runny yolk or until cooked to your liking. Remove from the pan using a slotted spoon. Serve each portion of hash topped with an egg.

Cauliflower rarebits

Ingredients

1 tbsp vegetable oil

1 large cauliflower, trimmed and sliced into 2 thick steaks through the root to hold shape (use the trimmings for another dish)

For the rarebit

20g butter

20g flour

100ml milk

100g grated extra mature cheddar

large pinch cayenne pepper

1 tbsp English mustard

large splash of Worcestershire sauce or vegetarian alternative

2 egg yolks

red onion chutney and a watercress salad, to serve

Preparation

STEP 1

Heat the oil in a large frying pan and sear the cauliflower steaks for 3-4 mins on each side until nicely browned. Lift onto kitchen paper, then put in the fridge to keep cool. Can be done up to two days ahead.

STEP 2

To make the rarebit, melt the butter in a saucepan and stir in the flour to make a sandy paste. Add the milk a little at a time to make a thick white sauce. Bubble gently, stirring often for a couple of mins, then stir in the cheese, cayenne, mustard and Worcestershire sauce and stir until the cheese has melted into a smooth, rich sauce. Remove the pan from the heat and leave to cool slightly, then beat in the yolks and season. Transfer to an airtight container and keep in the fridge if not using straight away. Can be made up to two days ahead.

STEP 3

Before you assemble, take the cheesy rarebit mix out of the fridge at least an hour before you need it. Heat oven to 190C/170C fan/gas 5. Lay the cauliflower on a baking sheet, then divide and spread or press on the rarebit mix until completely covered. Bake in the oven for 12-15 mins, then finish under a hot grill until bubbling and golden. Transfer the cauliflower rarebits to two plates and serve with a spoonful of chutney and a generous handful of watercress salad. Perfect with a pint of beer.

Potato scones with smoked salmon & soured cream

Ingredients

1 large Maris Piper potato (about 225g), quartered

2 tbsp unsalted butter, plus extra for frying

60g plain flour, plus extra for dusting

½ tsp baking powder

vegetable oil, for frying

100g smoked salmon or trout

60g soured cream

1 tbsp finely chopped chives

Preparation

STEP 1

Bring a small pan of water to the boil and simmer the potatoes for 12-15 mins until tender. Drain and leave to steam-dry. Return the potatoes to the pan and mash with the butter. Stir in the flour, baking powder, ½ tsp salt and a good grinding of black pepper.

STEP 2

Tip the potato mixture onto a lightly floured work surface and press into a circle roughly 15cm wide and about 1cm thick, then cut into four wedges.

STEP 3

Heat a splash of oil and a knob of butter in a non-stick skillet or frying pan over a medium heat, and fry one of the scones for 3-4 mins on each side until golden brown. Repeat with the remaining scones.

STEP 4

Divide the scones and smoked salmon or trout between two plates, then top with the soured cream and chopped chives. Season and serve.

Red velvet pancakes

Ingredients

200g self raising flour

2 tbsp cocoa powder

1 tsp baking powder

1 tbsp golden caster sugar

½ tsp vanilla extract

230ml milk

3 eggs

25g butter, melted plus extra for frying

red gel food colouring

For the toppings

100g cream cheese

4 tbsp maple syrup

100g chocolate chips

icing sugar, for dusting

handful blueberries (optional)

Preparation

STEP 1

Mix all of the pancake Ingredients (except the food colouring) together in a large bowl, whisk thoroughly until smooth. Now add a small amount of red food colouring and mix again. Add more colouring until the batter is a rich reddish brown.

STEP 2

Put a small knob of butter in a large non-stick frying pan over a medium-low heat and cook until melted and foaming. Pour 2 tbsp of the mixture into the pan and use the back of the spoon to shape it into a 8-9cm round disc. Depending on the size of your pan you may be able to get 2 or 3 pancakes to cook at the same time. Cook for 2-3 mins on the first side, then flip over and cook for another 1 min on the other.

STEP 3

Heat oven to its lowest setting and stack up the cooked pancakes on a baking tray to keep warm in the oven while you cook the rest. In a small bowl mix together the cream cheese and maple syrup then set aside until needed. To serve, stack the pancakes with the cream cheese mixture and chocolate chips in between them then finish with a final dollop of the cream cheese, a dusting of icing sugar and a few fresh blueberries if you like.

Buckwheat galettes

Ingredients

80g buckwheat flour

5 medium eggs

250ml milk

2 tsp Dijon mustard

4 tbsp single cream

100g mature gruyère, comté or cheddar, grated

butter, for frying

100g ham, torn

fried mushrooms or steamed spinach, to serve (optional)

Preparation

STEP 1

Mix the flour, 1 egg, the milk and a pinch of salt in a jug or bowl. Set aside for 30 mins, or up to 3 hrs. Mash together the mustard, cream and cheese in another bowl. Heat the oven to 200C/180C fan/gas 6, and line two baking trays with baking parchment or foil.

STEP 2

Melt the butter in a large frying pan, then once foaming, add enough batter to just cover the pan, swirling it to cover the surface in a thin layer (pour any excess back into the batter bowl). Cook until the surface is set and the underside is browning, carefully flip and cook for another minute or 2, then take off the heat.

STEP 3

Spoon a quarter of the cheese mixture onto the middle of the pancake, using the spoon to create space in the centre to hold an egg. Crack one into the space and lay a few pieces of ham around the edges. Fold each side of the pancake in towards the centre to make a square. Cook in the pan for another 30 secs-1 min, then transfer to a baking tray. Repeat with the rest of the pancakes, then bake for 6-7 mins until the egg whites are set. Serve with fried mushrooms or wilted spinach, if you like.

Nuts & seeds granola

Ingredients

150g rolled oats

150g mixed nuts (we used whole hazelnuts, flaked almonds and whole pecans)

50g mixed seeds (we used a mixed bag containing sunflower, pumpkin, hemp and golden linseed)

50g raisins

1 tsp ground cinnamon

¼ tsp sea salt

1 tsp almond extract (vanilla works well too, if you prefer)

50ml vegetable oil

100ml maple syrup

milk or yogurt, and fruit (optional), to serve

Preparation

STEP 1

Heat the oven to 180C/160C fan gas 4. Line a large baking sheet with baking parchment to prevent the granola from sticking. Put all of the dry Ingredients in a large mixing bowl. Whisk together the almond extract, vegetable oil and maple syrup in a jug, then pour into the bowl with the dry Ingredients.

STEP 2

Mix together well, making sure that all the dry Ingredients are well coated and that there are no dry bits. Tip the mixture onto the lined baking sheet and spread out in an even layer. Cook for about 25-30 mins until golden. You will need to give the mixture a few turns every 8-10 mins to make sure it dries out evenly and doesn't clump together too much. Keep an eye on it as nuts can burn easily.

STEP 3

Remove from the oven and leave to cool completely on the tray. Break up any large clumps of granola with a wooden spoon. Will keep for up to one month in an airtight container. Serve with milk or yogurt, and fresh seasonal fruit, if you like.

Pastrami-cured salmon

Ingredients

800g side of salmon (the freshest you can get)

250g coarse sea salt

100g light brown soft sugar

2 tbsp coriander seeds

1 tsp ground coriander

1 tbsp caraway seeds

1 tbsp black peppercorns

1 bay leaf

1 tsp sweet smoked paprika

½ tsp cayenne pepper

2 tbsp black treacle

To serve

soft cheese, rye bread or bagels, dill pickles and chopped dill

Preparation

STEP 1

Three days before you want to serve the salmon, put it, skin-side down, in a rimmed dish. Combine the salt and sugar, then set aside.

STEP 2

Fry the coriander seeds, ground coriander, caraway seeds and peppercorns in a small dry frying pan set over a medium heat for 2-3 mins. Tip into a spice grinder or small food processor along with the bay, and blitz until finely ground. Stir the spice mixture into the salt and sugar mix. Pat the spiced salt mixture all over and around the salmon so it's well packed onto the flesh. Wrap tightly in cling film, then set a plate or board and something heavy (such as a couple of cans) on top to weigh the fish down. Chill for 48 hrs.

STEP 3

Heat the paprika, cayenne and black treacle in a pan until loosened, then remove from the heat and leave to cool slightly until just warm. Brush the excess salt off the salmon and rinse the fish under cold running water. Pat dry with kitchen paper, then transfer to a clean dish. Brush with the warm treacle mixture until well coated (you may need to generously brush the fish several times before the coating covers the fish well), then wrap in a fresh sheet of cling film. Chill for another 24 hrs.

STEP 4

When you're ready to serve, set the salmon on a board and thinly slice with a sharp knife, avoiding the layer of skin at the bottom. Serve with soft cheese, rye bread or bagels, pickles and some chopped dill for everyone to help themselves.

Minty griddled chicken & peach salad

Ingredients

1 lime, zested and juiced

1 tbsp rapeseed oil

2 tbsp mint, finely chopped, plus a few leaves to serve

1 garlic clove, finely grated

2 skinless chicken breast fillets (300g)

160g fine beans, trimmed and halved

2 peaches (200g), each cut into 8 thick wedges

1 red onion, cut into wedges

1 large Little Gem lettuce (165g), roughly shredded

½ x 60g pack rocket

1 small avocado, stoned and sliced

240g cooked new potatoes

Preparation

STEP 1

Mix the lime zest and juice, oil and mint, then put half in a bowl with the garlic. Thickly slice the chicken at a slight angle, add to the garlic mixture and toss together with plenty of black pepper.

STEP 2

Cook the beans in a pan of water for 3-4 mins until just tender. Meanwhile, griddle the chicken and onion for a few mins each side until cooked and tender. Transfer to a plate, then quickly griddle the peaches. If you don't have a griddle pan, use a non-stick frying pan with a drop of oil.

STEP 3

Toss the warm beans and onion in the remaining mint mixture, and pile onto a platter or into individual shallow bowls with the lettuce and rocket. Top with the avocado, peaches and chicken and scatter over the mint. Serve with the potatoes while still warm.

Mexican-style bean soup with shredded chicken & lime

Ingredients

2 tsp rapeseed oil

1 large onion, finely chopped

1 red pepper, cut into chunks

2 garlic cloves, chopped

2 tsp mild chilli powder

1 tsp ground coriander

1 tsp ground cumin

400g can chopped tomatoes

400g can black beans

1 tsp vegetable bouillon powder

1 cooked skinless chicken breast, about 125g, shredded

handful chopped coriander

1 lime, juiced

½ red chilli, deseeded and finely chopped (optional)

Preparation

STEP 1

Heat the oil in a medium pan, add the onion and pepper, and fry, stirring frequently, for 10 mins. Stir in the garlic and spices, then tip in the tomatoes and beans with their liquid, half a can of water and the bouillon powder. Simmer, covered, for 15 mins.

STEP 2

Meanwhile, tip the chicken into a bowl, add the coriander and lime juice with a little chilli (if using, or see tip below for guacamole alternative) and toss well. Ladle the soup into two bowls, top with the chicken and serve.

Moroccan freekeh traybake

Ingredients

2 tbsp olive oil

400g can chickpeas, rinsed and drained

1 tsp ground coriander

1 tsp ground cumin

½ tsp chilli flakes

270g cherry tomatoes

½ x 400g can apricot halves, drained and roughly chopped

70g green olives

250g pouch cooked freekeh

70g fat-free Greek yogurt

small bunch dill, finely chopped

Preparation

STEP 1

Heat oven to 200C/180C fan/ gas 6. Toss the oil with the chickpeas, spices and chilli flakes in a medium roasting tin. Roast for 15 mins or until the chickpeas are beginning to crisp and turn golden brown. Add the tomatoes, apricots, olives and freekeh to the pan and toss everything together. Return to the oven for a final 10-15 mins until the tomatoes start to burst and everything is piping hot. Season to taste.

STEP 2

Combine the yogurt and most of the dill and season with salt. Serve the freekeh with any extra dill fronds scattered over and a dollop of the herby yogurt.

Healthy chicken burritos

Ingredients

2 tsp rapeseed oil

1 large red pepper, halved lengthways, deseeded and cut into thick strips

1 tsp cumin seeds

2-3 tsp mild chilli powder, to taste

400g can black beans

198g can sweetcorn, drained

1 tbsp tomato purée

1 large garlic clove, finely grated

220g pouch cooked wholegrain rice (or leftover cooked brown rice)

300g cooked chicken, sliced or shredded (or a combination of leg and breast meat left over from a roast)

15g coriander, chopped

2 small avocados, stoned and quartered

1 lime, juiced

4 large wholemeal tortilla wraps

Preparation

STEP 1

Heat the oil in a large non-stick frying pan and cook the pepper, covered, for 10 mins over a low heat until softened and lightly charred.

STEP 2

Meanwhile, in a dry frying pan, toast the spices gently over a low heat for 2-3 mins until fragrant, then tip in the beans, along with their liquid, the sweetcorn, tomato purée and garlic. Mix well and turn the heat up to medium so the mixture bubbles, then stir in the rice, chicken and coriander. Cook for 3-4 mins until piping hot. Will keep chilled for up to a day. Leave to cool completely first. Reheat in a pan or the microwave until piping hot.

STEP 3

Toss the avocado in a bowl with the lime juice. Lay the tortillas out on a work surface and pile the rice down the centre leaving a space at either side. Top with the peppers and avocado, then fold up the tortillas at each end to enclose the filling and tightly roll up the wrap. Put in the pan that you cooked the peppers in, seam-side down, and cook gently on each side over a low heat to lightly toast, about 2-3 mins. You may need to do this in batches.

DELICIOUS POTS SYNDROME DIET LUNCH RECIPES

Roasted pepper sauce for pasta or chicken

Ingredients

3 red peppers

2 peeled red onions

1 tbsp oil

½ tsp dried thyme

500g passata

Preparation

STEP 1

Heat oven to 220C/fan 200C/gas 7. Cut the peppers and the onions into chunks. Toss in the oil and dried thyme, then roast for 30 mins until soft and slightly blackened.

STEP 2

Cool, then blend or process until just chunky. Stir through the passata, season and warm through.

Thirty-minute courgettes with dukkah sprinkle

Ingredients

1 tbsp rapeseed oil

2 onions, halved and sliced

2 tsp ground coriander

2 tsp smoked paprika

400g can chopped tomatoes

2 tsp vegetable bouillon powder

2 large courgettes, sliced

400g can butter beans, drained

180g cherry tomatoes

160g frozen peas

15g coriander, chopped

For the dukkah

1 tsp coriander seeds

1 tsp cumin seeds

1 tbsp sesame seeds

25g flaked almonds

Preparation

STEP 1

Heat the oil in a large non-stick pan and fry the onions for 5 mins, stirring occasionally until starting to colour. Stir in the ground coriander and paprika, then tip in the tomatoes with a can of water. Add the bouillon powder and courgettes, cover and cook for 6 mins.

STEP 2

Meanwhile, make the dukkah. Warm the whole spices, sesame seeds and almonds in a pan until aromatic, stirring frequently, then remove the pan from the heat.

STEP 3

Add the butter beans, tomatoes and peas to the courgettes, cover and cook for 5 mins more. Stir in the coriander, then spoon into bowls. Crush the spices and almonds using a pestle and mortar and scatter on top. If you're cooking for two people, put half the seed mix in a jar and chill half the veg for another day.

Herby broccoli & pea soup

Ingredients

1 tbsp rapeseed oil

1 onion, finely chopped

1 large garlic clove, crushed

400g broccoli, chopped into small florets

300g frozen peas

200g chard, chopped

1l low-salt veg stock

½ small bunch of basil, chopped

small bunch of dill, chopped

1 lemon, zested and juiced

2 tbsp pumpkin seeds, toasted

Preparation

STEP 1

Heat the oil in a large saucepan. Add the onion and fry for 8 mins until soft and translucent. Add the garlic and cook for 1 min more. Tip in the broccoli, peas and chard, then pour over the stock and bring the mixture to the boil. Reduce the heat to a simmer, cover and cook for 25 mins.

STEP 2

Stir through the herbs, lemon zest and juice, then blitz the soup with a stick blender until completely smooth. Ladle into bowls and serve with the toasted pumpkin seeds scattered over the top.

Chicken & tzatziki wraps

Ingredients

1 cucumber, three-quarters deseeded and coarsely grated, the rest halved and sliced

250g Greek yogurt

500g chicken breast, thinly sliced

2tbsp olive oil

4 wholemeal wraps

4 large ripe tomatoes, thinly sliced

Preparation

STEP 1

For the tzatziki, tip the grated cucumber and yogurt into a bowl, mix well and season. Set aside. Season the chicken with salt and pepper and rub with 1 tbsp of the olive oil. Heat the remaining oil in a pan over a medium heat. Cook the chicken for 8-10 mins until cooked through and golden brown.

STEP 2

Warm the wraps in a dry pan or microwave. Spread 2 tbsp of the tzatziki onto each wrap, top with the

chicken, tomatoes and sliced cucumber. Season
with a little more pepper, if you like, then fold the
sides of the wrap over the filling, roll up tightly and
serve.

Minestrone in minutes

Ingredients

1l hot vegetable stock

400g tin chopped tomato

100g thin spaghetti, broken into short lengths

350g frozen mixed vegetable

4 tbsp pesto

drizzle of olive oil

coarsely grated vegetarian parmesan-style cheese, to serve

Preparation

STEP 1

Bring the stock to the boil with the tomatoes, then add the spaghetti and cook for 6 mins or until done. A few minutes before the pasta is ready, add the vegetables and bring back to the boil. Simmer for 2 mins until everything is cooked.

STEP 2

Serve in bowls drizzled with pesto and oil, sprinkled with parmesan.

Red lentil soup

Ingredients

1 white onion, finely sliced

2 tsp olive oil

3 garlic cloves, sliced

2 carrots, scrubbed and diced

85g red lentils

1 vegetable stock cube, crumbled

generous sprigs parsley, chopped (about 2 tbsp) plus a few extra leaves

Preparation

STEP 1

Put the kettle on to boil while you finely slice the onion. Heat the oil in a medium pan, add the onion and fry for 2 mins while you slice the garlic and dice the carrots. Add them to the pan, and cook briefly over the heat.

STEP 2

Pour in 1 litre of the boiling water from the kettle, stir in the lentils and stock cube, then cover the pan and cook over a medium heat for 15 mins until the lentils are tender. Take off the heat and stir in the parsley. Ladle into bowls, and scatter with extra parsley leaves, if you like.

Prosciutto, kale & butter bean stew

Ingredients

80g pack prosciutto, torn into pieces

2 tbsp olive oil

1 fennel bulb, sliced

2 garlic clove, crushed

1 tsp chilli flakes

4 thyme sprigs

150ml white wine or chicken stock

2 x 400g cans butter beans

400g can cherry tomatoes

200g bag sliced kale

Preparation

STEP 1

Fry the prosciutto in a dry saucepan over a high heat until crisp, then remove half with a slotted spoon and set aside. Turn the heat down to low, pour in the oil and tip in the fennel with a pinch of salt. Cook for 5 mins until softened, then throw in the garlic, chilli flakes and thyme and cook for a further 2 mins, then pour in the wine or stock and bring to a simmer.

STEP 2

Tip both cans of butter beans into the stew, along with their liquid, then add the tomatoes, season well and bring everything to a simmer. Cook, undisturbed, for 5 mins, then stir through the kale. Once wilted, ladle the stew into bowls, removing the thyme sprigs and topping each portion with the remaining prosciutto.

Lighter chicken tacos

Ingredients

For the chicken

2 tsp rapeseed oil

1 tsp ground cumin

1 tsp smoked paprika

450g skinless chicken breasts, preferably organic

For the salsa

4 medium tomatoes, preferably on the vine, halved

1 red pepper, quartered

1 small red onion, cut into 8 wedges

¼ tsp rapeseed oil

2 tsp lime juice

¼ tsp ground cumin

good pinch of chilli flakes

For the guacamole

2 medium-sized ripe avocados, stoned, peeled and
roughly chopped

4 tsp lime juice

2 spring onions, ends trimmed, finely chopped

3 tbsp chopped coriander

good pinch of chilli flakes

To serve

8 corn tacos shells

8 tsp 0% Greek yogurt

2 Little Gem lettuces, shredded

chopped coriander

lime wedges, for squeezing over

Preparation

STEP 1

Mix the oil with the cumin and paprika on a large plate. Sit the chicken on the plate and rub the spiced oil all over it. Season with pepper and a pinch of salt, then cover and set aside while you prepare the salsa.

STEP 2

Heat the grill to high for 10 mins. Meanwhile, line a large baking tray with foil and lay the tomatoes (cut-side up) on it, along with the pepper and red onion. Brush the oil over the onion, and season the tomatoes and onion with pepper. Grill for 12-15 mins, turning the tomatoes and onion halfway through, until well charred. Remove (leaving the grill on) and set aside to cool – put the pepper in a bowl and cover with cling film so that it's easier to skin later.

STEP 3

For the guacamole, put the avocado in a bowl and briefly mash with a fork, leaving some chunky pieces for texture. Gently mix in the lime juice, spring onions, coriander and chilli flakes. Season with pepper and a pinch of salt.

STEP 4

Re-line the baking tray with foil and lay the chicken on it, plump-side up. Grill for about 10 mins until cooked – there is no need to turn it. Meanwhile, scoop out and discard as much of the seeds and juice from the tomatoes as you can (so the salsa isn't too wet), leaving the pulp and charred skin. When the pepper is cool enough to handle, peel off and discard the skin. Chop the tomatoes and onion, and dice the pepper. Combine in a bowl with the lime juice, cumin, chilli flakes, some pepper and a pinch of salt.

STEP 5

When the chicken is cooked, remove from the grill, cover loosely with foil and set aside for 5 mins.

STEP 6

Heat oven to 180C/160C fan/gas 4. Cut the chicken into chunky slices and spoon over the juices. When ready to serve, lay the taco shells on a baking sheet and warm through for 2-3 mins. Serve the chicken, taco shells, yogurt, lettuce, coriander and lime wedges in separate bowls, so that everyone can build their own tacos.

Bombay potato frittata

Ingredients

4 new potatoes, sliced into 5mm rounds

100g baby spinach, chopped

1 tbsp rapeseed oil

1 onion, halved and sliced

1 large garlic clove, finely grated

½ tsp ground coriander

½ tsp ground cumin

¼ tsp black mustard seeds

¼ tsp turmeric

3 tomatoes, roughly chopped

2 large eggs

½ green chilli, deseeded and finely chopped

1 small bunch of coriander, finely chopped

1 tbsp mango chutney

3 tbsp fat-free Greek yogurt

Preparation

STEP 1

Cook the potatoes in a pan of boiling water for 6 mins, or until tender. Drain and leave to steam-dry. Meanwhile, put the spinach in a heatproof bowl with 1 tbsp water. Cover and microwave for 3 mins on high, or until wilted.

STEP 2

Heat the rapeseed oil in a medium non-stick frying pan. Add the onion and cook over a medium heat for 10 mins until golden and sticky. Stir in the garlic, ground coriander, ground cumin, mustard seeds and turmeric, and cook for 1 min more. Add the tomatoes and wilted spinach and cook for another 3 mins, then add the potatoes.

STEP 3

Heat the grill to medium. Lightly beat the eggs with the chilli and most of the fresh coriander and pour over the potato mixture. Grill for 4-5 mins, or until golden and just set, with a very slight wobble in the middle.

STEP 4

Leave to cool, then slice into wedges. Mix the mango chutney, yogurt and remaining fresh coriander together. Serve with the frittata wedges.

Chunky butternut mulligatawny

Ingredients

2 tbsp olive or rapeseed oil

2 onions, finely chopped

2 dessert apples, peeled and finely chopped

3 celery sticks, finely chopped

½ small butternut squash, peeled, seeds removed, chopped into small pieces

2-3 heaped tbsp gluten-free curry powder (depending on how spicy you like it)

1 tbsp ground cinnamon

1 tbsp nigella seeds (also called black onion or kalonji seeds)

2 x 400g cans chopped tomatoes

1 ½l gluten-free chicken or vegetable stock

140g basmati rice

small pack parsley, chopped

3 tbsp mango chutney, plus a little to serve, if you like (optional)

natural yogurt, to serve

Preparation

STEP 1

Heat the oil in your largest saucepan. Add the onions, apples and celery with a pinch of salt. Cook for 10 mins, stirring now and then, until softened. Add the butternut squash, curry powder, cinnamon, nigella seeds and a grind of black pepper. Cook for 2 mins more, then stir in the tomatoes and stock. Cover with a lid and simmer for 15 mins.

STEP 2

By now the vegetables should be tender but not mushy. Stir in the rice, pop the lid back on and simmer for another 12 mins until the rice is cooked through. Taste and add more seasoning if needed. Stir through the parsley and mango chutney, then serve in bowls with yogurt and extra mango chutney on top, if you like.

Red lentil & chorizo soup

Ingredients

1 tbsp olive oil, plus extra for drizzling

200g cooking chorizo, peeled and diced

1 large onion, chopped

2 carrots, chopped

pinch of cumin seeds

3 garlic cloves, chopped

1 tsp smoked paprika, plus extra for sprinkling

pinch of golden caster sugar

small splash red wine vinegar

250g red lentil

2 x 400g cans chopped tomato

850ml chicken stock

plain yogurt, to serve

Preparation

STEP 1

Heat the oil in a large pan. Add the chorizo and cook until crisp and it has released its oils. Remove with a slotted spoon into a bowl, leaving the fat in the pan. Fry the onion, carrots and cumin seeds for 10 mins until soft and glistening, then add the garlic and fry for 1 min more. Scatter over the paprika and sugar, cook for 1 min, then splash in the vinegar. Simmer for a moment, then stir in the lentils, and pour over the tomatoes and chicken stock.

STEP 2

Give it a good stir, then simmer for 30 mins or until the lentils are tender. Blitz with a hand blender until smooth-ish but still chunky. Can be made several days ahead or frozen for 6 months at this point. Serve in bowls, drizzled with yogurt and olive oil, scattered with the chorizo and a sprinkling of paprika.

Baked salmon

Ingredients

4 skinless salmon fillets

1 tbsp olive oil or melted butter

chopped herbs, lemon slices and steamed long-stem broccoli, to serve (optional)

Preparation

STEP 1

Heat the oven to 180C/160C fan/gas 4. Brush each salmon fillet with the oil or butter and season well.

STEP 2

Put the salmon fillets in an ovenproof dish. Cover if you prefer your salmon to be tender, or leave uncovered if you want the flesh to roast slightly.

STEP 3

Roast for 10-15 mins (or about 4 mins per 1cm thickness) until just opaque and easily flaked with a fork. Serve with a sprinkling of chopped herbs, lemon slices and steamed long-stem broccoli, if you like.

Carrot & ginger soup

Ingredients

1 tbsp rapeseed oil

1 large onion, chopped

2 tbsp coarsely grated ginger

2 garlic cloves, sliced

½ tsp ground nutmeg

850ml vegetable stock

500g carrot (preferably organic), sliced

400g can cannellini beans (no need to drain)

Supercharged topping

4 tbsp almonds in their skins, cut into slivers

sprinkle of nutmeg

Preparation

STEP 1

Heat the oil in a large pan, add the onion, ginger and garlic, and fry for 5 mins until starting to soften. Stir in the nutmeg and cook for 1 min more.

STEP 2

Pour in the stock, add the carrots, beans and their liquid, then cover and simmer for 20-25 mins until the carrots are tender.

STEP 3

Scoop a third of the mixture into a bowl and blitz the remainder with a hand blender or in a food processor until smooth. Return everything to the pan and heat until bubbling. Serve topped with the almonds and nutmeg.

Healthy egg & chips

Ingredients

500g potatoes, diced

2 shallots, sliced

1 tbsp olive oil

2 tsp dried crushed oregano or 1 tsp fresh leaves

200g small mushroom

4 eggs

Preparation

STEP 1

Heat oven to 200C/fan 180C/gas 6. Tip the potatoes and shallots into a large, non-stick roasting tin, drizzle with the oil, sprinkle over the oregano, then mix everything together well. Bake for 40-45 mins (or until starting to go brown), add the mushrooms, then cook for a further 10 mins until the potatoes are browned and tender.

STEP 2

Make four gaps in the vegetables and crack an egg into each space. Return to the oven for 3-4 mins or until the eggs are cooked to your liking.

DELICIOUS POTS SYNDROME DIET DINNER RECIPES

Pasta primavera

Ingredients

75g young broad beans (use frozen if you can't get fresh)

2 x 100g pack asparagus tips

170g peas (use frozen if you can't get fresh)

350g spaghetti or tagliatelle

175g pack baby leeks, trimmed and sliced

1 tbsp olive oil, plus extra to serve

1 tbsp butter

200ml tub fromage frais or creme fraiche

handful fresh chopped herbs (we used mint, parsley and chives)

parmesan (or vegetarian alternative), shaved, to serve

Preparation

STEP 1

Bring a pan of salted water to the boil and put a steamer (or colander) over the water. Steam the beans, asparagus and peas until just tender, then set aside. Boil the pasta following pack instructions.

STEP 2

Meanwhile, fry the leeks gently in the oil and butter for 5 mins or until soft. Add the fromage frais to the leeks and very gently warm through, stirring constantly to ensure it doesn't split. Add the herbs

and steamed vegetables with a splash of pasta water
to loosen.

STEP 3

Drain the pasta and stir into the sauce. Adjust the
seasoning, then serve scattered with the cheese and
drizzled with a little extra olive oil.

Pot-roast beef with French onion gravy

Ingredients

1kg silverside or topside of beef with no added fat

2 tbsp olive oil

8 young carrots, tops trimmed (but leave a little, if you like)

1 celery stick, finely chopped

200ml white wine

600ml rich beef stock

2 bay leaves

500g onion

a few thyme sprigs

1 tsp butter

1 tsp light brown or light muscovado sugar

2 tsp plain flour

Preparation

STEP 1

Heat oven to 160C/140C fan/gas 3. Rub the meat with 1 tsp of the oil and plenty of seasoning. Heat a large flameproof casserole dish and brown the meat all over for about 10 mins. Meanwhile, add 2 tsp oil to a frying pan and fry the carrots and celery for 10 mins until turning golden.

STEP 2

Lift the beef onto a plate, splash the wine into the hot casserole and boil for 2 mins. Pour in the stock, return the beef, then tuck in the carrots, celery and bay leaves, trying not to submerge the carrots too much. Cover and cook in the oven for 2 hrs. (I like to turn the beef halfway through cooking.)

STEP 3

Meanwhile, thinly slice the onions. Heat 1 tbsp oil in a pan and stir in the onions, thyme and some seasoning. Cover and cook gently for 20 mins until the onions are softened but not coloured. Remove the lid, turn up the heat, add the butter and sugar, then let the onions caramelise to a dark golden brown, stirring often. Remove the thyme sprigs, then set aside.

STEP 4

When the beef is ready, it will be tender and easy to pull apart at the edges. Remove it from the casserole and snip off the strings. Reheat the onion pan, stir in the flour and cook for 1 min. Whisk the floury onions into the beefy juices in the casserole, to make a thick onion gravy. Taste for seasoning. Add the beef and carrots back to the casserole, or slice the beef and bring to the table on a platter, with the carrots to the side and the gravy spooned over.

Chicken tacos

Ingredients

250g plain flour, plus extra for dusting

2 tbsp rapeseed oil

2 tbsp taco or fajita seasoning (see tip, below)

5-6 skinless chicken breasts, sliced

¼ red cabbage, finely shredded

3 limes, 1 juiced, 2 cut into wedges

small bunch of coriander, chopped

4 sweetcorn cob, kernels sliced off, or 400g frozen sweetcorn

400g can black beans, drained and rinsed

2 garlic cloves, crushed

4 tbsp fat-free yogurt, to serve

chilli sauce, to serve

Preparation

STEP 1

Combine the flour with half the oil and a small pinch of salt in a bowl. Pour over 125-150ml warm water, then bring together into a soft dough with your hands. Cut into six equal pieces, then cut four of the pieces in half again, so you have eight small pieces and two large. Roll all the pieces out on a floured work surface until they're as thin as you can get them.

STEP 2

Heat a dry frying pan over a medium-high heat and cook the small and large tortillas for 2-3 mins on each side until golden and toasted (do this one at a time). Leave the large tortillas to cool, then cover and reserve for use in the lunchboxes (see tip below). Keep the small tortillas warm in foil.

STEP 3

Sprinkle the taco seasoning over the chicken in a bowl, and toss to combine. Toss the cabbage with the lime juice, half the coriander and some seasoning in another bowl, then leave to pickle.

STEP 4

Meanwhile, heat two frying pans over a high heat. Divide the remaining oil between the pans and fry the sweetcorn and a pinch of salt until sizzling and turning golden, stirring occasionally – you want the sweetcorn to char slightly, as this adds flavour, so you may need to leave it to cook undisturbed for a bit. While the sweetcorn cooks and chars, fry the chicken in the larger pan until cooked through and golden (you may need to do this in batches).

STEP 5

Tip the black beans and garlic into the sweetcorn and stir to warm through. Squeeze over two of the lime wedges.

STEP 6

Reserve two spoonfuls each of the chicken (about 1 chicken breast) and sweetcorn mix for use in the lunchboxes (see tip, below), then serve the rest in bowls alongside the cabbage, yogurt, lime wedges, remaining coriander, chilli sauce and tortillas for everyone to dig into.

Chicken with crushed harissa chickpeas

Ingredients

2 tbsp rapeseed oil

1 onion, chopped

1 red pepper, finely sliced

1 yellow pepper, finely sliced

4 chicken breasts

1 tbsp za'atar

400g can chickpeas

1½ tbsp red harissa paste

150g baby spinach

½ small bunch of parsley, finely chopped

lemon wedges, to serve

Preparation

STEP 1

Heat 1 tbsp of oil in a frying pan over a medium heat and fry the onions and peppers for 7 mins until softened and golden.

STEP 2

Meanwhile, put the chicken between two sheets of baking parchment and lightly bash until about 2cm thick. Mix together the remaining oil and the za'atar, then rub over the chicken. Season to taste.

STEP 3

Heat the grill to high. Put the chicken on a baking tray lined with foil, and grill for 3-4 mins each side, or until golden and cooked through.

STEP 4

Heat the chickpeas in a pan with the harissa paste and 2 tbsp water until warmed through, then roughly mash with a potato masher. Wilt the spinach in a pan with 1 tbsp of water or in the microwave in a heatproof bowl. Stir the pepper and onion mixture, spinach and parsley through the chickpeas. Serve with the sliced chicken and the lemon wedges for squeezing over.

Sardine tomato pasta with gremolata

Ingredients

75g wholemeal spaghetti

½ x 120g can sardines in oil

½ tbsp capers, drained

2 garlic cloves, crushed

2 tomatoes, roughly chopped

30g rocket

½ lemon, zested

small handful of parsley, finely chopped

Preparation

STEP 1

Cook the pasta following pack instructions in a large pan of boiling salted water. Heat 1 tbsp oil from the can of sardines in a non-stick frying pan over a medium heat and sizzle the capers and half the garlic for 1-2 mins until fragrant. Tip in the tomatoes and fry for 4-5 mins more until softened and bursting. Stir in the sardines and rocket, tossing a few times to break up the fish and wilt the leaves. Season.

STEP 2

For the gremolata, combine the lemon zest, parsley and remaining garlic in a small bowl, and season. Drain the pasta and top with the sardine sauce and gremolata.

Winter vegetable & lentil soup

Ingredients

85g dried red lentils

2 carrots, quartered lengthways then diced

3 sticks celery, sliced

2 small leeks, sliced

2 tbsp tomato purée

1 tbsp fresh thyme leaves

3 large garlic cloves, chopped

1 tbsp vegetable bouillon powder

1 heaped tsp ground coriander

Preparation

STEP 1

Tip all the Ingredients into a large pan. Pour over 1½ litres boiling water, then stir well.

STEP 2

Cover and leave to simmer for 30 mins until the vegetables and lentils are tender.

STEP 3

Ladle into bowls and eat straightaway, or if you like a really thick texture, blitz a third of the soup with a hand blender or in a food processor.

Vegan chickpea curry jacket potatoes

Ingredients

4 sweet potatoes

1 tbsp coconut oil

1 ½ tsp cumin seeds

1 large onion, diced

2 garlic cloves, crushed

thumb-sized piece ginger, finely grated

1 green chilli, finely chopped

1 tsp garam masala

1 tsp ground coriander

½ tsp turmeric

2 tbsp tikka masala paste

2 x 400g can chopped tomatoes

2 x 400g can chickpeas, drained

lemon wedges and coriander leaves, to serve

Preparation

STEP 1

Heat oven to 200C/180C fan/gas 6. Prick the sweet potatoes all over with a fork, then put on a baking tray and roast in the oven for 45 mins or until tender when pierced with a knife.

STEP 2

Meanwhile, melt the coconut oil in a large saucepan over medium heat. Add the cumin seeds and fry for 1 min until fragrant, then add the onion and fry for 7-10 mins until softened.

STEP 3

Put the garlic, ginger and green chilli into the pan, and cook for 2-3 mins. Add the spices and tikka masala paste and cook for a further 2 mins until fragrant, then tip in the tomatoes. Bring to a simmer, then tip in the chickpeas and cook for a further 20 mins until thickened. Season.

STEP 4

Put the roasted sweet potatoes on four plates and cut open lengthways. Spoon over the chickpea curry and squeeze over the lemon wedges. Season, then scatter with coriander before serving.

Salmon & ginger fish cakes

Ingredients

1 large sweet potato, cut into chips

4 tsp olive oil

2 x 140g/5oz skinless salmon fillets

thumbnail-size piece ginger, grated

zest 1 lime, plus wedges to serve

½ bunch spring onions, finely chopped

2 tbsp mayonnaise mixed with wasabi (optional)

Preparation

STEP 1

Heat oven to 200C/180C fan/gas 6. Toss the chips in a roasting tin with 1 tsp oil. Season and bake for 20-25 mins.

STEP 2

Chop the salmon as finely as you can and place in a bowl with the ginger, lime zest and seasoning. Heat 1 tsp oil in a non-stick pan and soften the spring onions for 2 mins. Stir into the salmon, mix well and shape into 4 patties.

STEP 3

Heat remaining oil in the pan and cook the patties for 3-4 mins each side until golden and cooked through. Cover with a lid and leave to rest for a few mins. Serve 2 patties each with the chips, mayo and lime wedges for squeezing.

Chipotle chicken

Ingredients

1 onion, chopped

1 garlic clove, sliced

2 tbsp sunflower oil

1-2 tbsp chipotle paste (see tip, below)

400g can chopped tomatoes

1 tbsp cider vinegar

8 skinless chicken thigh fillets

small bunch coriander, chopped

soured cream and rice, to serve

Preparation

STEP 1

Fry the onion and garlic in the oil in a deep, wide frying pan until soft. Add the chipotle paste (use 1 tbsp for a mild flavour and 2 tbsp for a hotter, stronger one). Stir and cook for 1 min, then add the tomatoes and cider vinegar. Bring to a simmer and cook for 10 mins with the lid half on. Stir to make sure it doesn't get too dry.

STEP 2

Add the chicken and cook for 10 mins or until cooked through, turning once. Scatter with coriander and serve with rice and soured cream.

Spaghetti with sardines

Ingredients

400g spaghetti

1 tbsp olive oil

2 garlic cloves, crushed

pinch chilli flakes

227g can chopped tomato

2 cans skinless and boneless sardines in tomato sauce

100g pitted black olives, roughly chopped

1 tbsp capers, drained

small handful parsley, chopped

Preparation

STEP 1

Cook the spaghetti in a large pan of boiling salted water according to pack instructions. Meanwhile, make the sauce. Heat the oil in a medium pan and cook the garlic for 1 min. Add the chilli flakes, tomatoes and sardines, breaking up roughly with a wooden spoon. Heat for 2-3 mins, then stir in the olives, capers and most of the parsley. Mix well to combine.

STEP 2

Drain the pasta, reserving a couple of tbsp of the water. Add the pasta to the sauce and mix well, adding the reserved water if the sauce is a little thick. Divide between 4 bowls and sprinkle with the remaining parsley.

Tuna, asparagus & white bean salad

Ingredients

1 large bunch asparagus

2 x cans tuna steaks in water, drained

2 x cans cannellini beans in water, drained

1 red onion, very finely chopped

2 tbsp capers

1 tbsp olive oil

1 tbsp red wine vinegar

2 tbsp tarragon, finely chopped

Preparation

STEP 1

Cook the asparagus in a large pan of boiling water for 4-5 mins until tender. Drain well, cool under running water, then cut into finger-length pieces. Toss together the tuna, beans, onion, capers and asparagus in a large serving bowl.

STEP 2

Mix the oil, vinegar and tarragon together, then pour over the salad. Chill until ready to serve.

Quick chicken hummus bowl

Ingredients

200g hummus

1 small lemon, zested and juiced

200g pouch cooked mixed grains

150g baby spinach, roughly chopped

1 small avocado, halved and sliced

1cooked chicken breast, sliced at an angle

100g pomegranate seeds

½ red onion, finely sliced

2 tbsp toasted almonds

Preparation

STEP 1

Mix 2 tbsp of the hummus with half the lemon juice, the lemon zest and enough water to make a drizzly dressing. Squeeze the grain pouch to separate the grains, then divide between two shallow bowls and toss through the dressing. Top each bowl with a handful of the spinach.

STEP 2

Squeeze the remaining lemon juice over the avocado halves, then add one half to each bowl. Divide the chicken, pomegranate seeds, onion, almonds and remaining hummus between the two bowls and gently mix everything together just before eating.

Broccoli pesto & pancetta pasta

Ingredients

300g head broccoli, broken into florets

300g pasta (we used orecchiette)

1 tbsp pine nuts

1 large bunch of basil

1 large garlic clove

2 tbsp parmesan, finely grated

1 tbsp olive oil

50g smoked pancetta, diced

200g cherry tomatoes, halved

Preparation

STEP 1

Bring a pan of lightly salted water to the boil. Add the broccoli and boil for 5 mins. Scoop out with a slotted spoon and set aside.

STEP 2

Put the pasta in the same pan and cook following pack instructions. Meanwhile, tip the broccoli into a food processor with the pine nuts, basil, garlic, parmesan and oil, and blitz until smooth. Season with black pepper and a little salt (the pancetta is very salty).

STEP 3

Set a frying pan over a medium heat and cook the pancetta for 2 mins. Add the tomatoes and cook for 3 mins, or until softened. Toss the pasta with the broccoli pesto, tomatoes and pancetta, and loosen with a splash of pasta water, if needed. Spoon into bowls and serve.

Pearl barley, bacon & leek casserole

Ingredients

1 tbsp olive oil

2 leeks, thickly sliced

2 garlic cloves, finely chopped

300g pearl barley, soaked for 1 hr

4 carrots, cubed

1 tbsp Dijon mustard, plus extra to serve

1l chicken stock

300g Savoy cabbage, shredded

200g lean bacon joint, cooked, chopped into small pieces

Preparation

STEP 1

Heat a large pan over a medium heat. Add the olive oil and cook the leeks for a few mins, then add the garlic and cook for just 1 min more.

STEP 2

Add the pearl barley, carrots and mustard, then pour over the chicken stock. Season with plenty of ground black pepper and simmer for 20 mins, stirring occasionally. Add the cabbage with the bacon, and cook for 5-10 mins until cabbage is wilted and tender. Serve with extra Dijon mustard on the side.

Crispy grilled feta with saucy butter beans

Ingredients

500ml passata

2 x 400g cans butter beans, drained and rinsed

2 garlic cloves, crushed

1 tsp dried oregano, plus a pinch

200g spinach

2 roasted red peppers, sliced

½ lemon, zested and juiced

100g block of feta, cut into chunks

½ tsp olive oil

4 small pittas

Preparation

STEP 1

Put a large ovenproof frying pan over a medium-high heat, and tip in the passata, butter beans, garlic, oregano, spinach and peppers. Stir together and cook for 6-8 mins until the sauce is bubbling and the spinach has wilted. Season, then add the lemon juice.

STEP 2

Heat the grill to high. Scatter the feta over the sauce, so it's still exposed, drizzle with the olive oil and sprinkle over the lemon zest plus a pinch of oregano, then grind over some black pepper. Grill for 5-8 mins until the feta is golden and crisp at the edges.

STEP 3

Meanwhile, toast the pittas under the grill or in the toaster, then serve with the beans and feta.

Vegetarian ramen

Ingredients

80g pack instant noodles (look for an Asian brand with a flavour like sesame)

2 spring onions, finely chopped

½ head pak choi

1 egg

1 tsp sesame seeds

chilli sauce, to serve

Preparation

STEP 1

Cook the noodles with the sachet of flavouring provided (or use stock instead of the sachet, if you have it). Add the spring onions and pak choi for the final min.

STEP 2

Meanwhile, simmer the egg for 6 mins from boiling, run it under cold water to stop it cooking, then peel it. Toast the sesame seeds in a frying pan.

STEP 3

Tip the noodles and greens into a deep bowl, halve the boiled egg and place on top. Sprinkle with sesame seeds, then drizzle with the sauce or sesame oil provided with the noodles, and chilli sauce, if using.

Baked cod

Ingredients

3 tbsp plain flour

4 cod loin fillets

2 tbsp olive oil

1 lemon, sliced

½ small bunch of thyme

Preparation

STEP 1

Heat the oven to 220C/200C fan/gas 7. Tip the flour into a bowl and add some seasoning. Turn each cod fillet in the flour until evenly coated.

STEP 2

Heat half the oil in a non-stick frying pan over a medium-high heat. Add the cod and fry on each side for 2 mins or until golden brown.

STEP 3

Transfer the cod to a roasting tin. Arrange the lemon slices and thyme on and around the fish and drizzle with the remaining oil. Bake for 10 mins or until cooked through.

Zesty haddock with crushed potatoes & peas

Ingredients

600g floury potato, unpeeled, cut into chunks

140g frozen peas

2 ½ tbsp extra-virgin olive oil

juice and zest ½ lemon

1 tbsp capers, roughly chopped

2 tbsp snipped chives

4 haddock or other chunky white fish fillets, about 120g each (or use 2 small per person)

2 tbsp plain flour

broccoli, to serve

Preparation

STEP 1

Cover the potatoes in cold water, bring to the boil, then turn to a simmer. Cook for 10 mins until tender, adding peas for the final min of cooking. Drain and roughly crush together, adding plenty of seasoning and 1 tbsp oil. Keep warm.

STEP 2

Meanwhile, for the dressing, mix 1 tbsp oil, the lemon juice and zest, capers and chives with some seasoning.

STEP 3

Dust the fish in the flour, tapping off any excess and season. Heat remaining oil in a non-stick frying pan. Fry the fish for 2-3 mins on each side until cooked, then add the dressing and warm through. Serve with the crush and broccoli.

DELICIOUS POTS SYNDROME DIET SNACK RECIPES

Spinach & sweet potato tortilla

Ingredients

300g bag baby spinach leaves

8 tbsp light olive oil

2 large onions, thinly sliced

4 medium sweet potatoes (800g/ 1lb 12oz), peeled, cut into thin slices

2 garlic cloves, finely chopped

8 large eggs

Preparation

STEP 1

Put the spinach in a large colander and pour over a kettleful of boiling water. Drain well and, when cooled a little, squeeze dry, trying not to mush up the spinach too much.

STEP 2

Heat 3 tbsp oil in a 25cm non-stick pan with a lid, then sweat the onions for 15 mins until really soft but not coloured. Add another 3 tbsp oil and add the potatoes and garlic. Mix in with the onions, season well, cover and cook over a gentle heat for another 15 mins or so until the potatoes are very tender. Stir occasionally to stop them catching.

STEP 3

Whisk the eggs in a large bowl, tip in the cooked potato and onion, and mix together. Separate the spinach clumps, add to the mix and fold through, trying not to break up the potato too much.

STEP 4

Add 2 tbsp more oil to the pan and pour in the sweet potato and egg mix. Cover and cook over a low-medium heat for 20 mins until the base and sides are golden brown and the centre has mostly set. Run a palette knife around the sides to stop it from sticking. 5 To turn the tortilla over, put a plate face down onto the pan, then flip it over. Slide the tortilla back into the pan and cook for a further 5-10 mins until just set and golden all over. (Don't worry if it breaks up a little on the edges as you're turning it – it will look perfect when it's cooked through and set.) Continue cooking on the other side until just set and golden all over. Again use a palette knife to release the tortilla from the sides.

Allow to rest for 5 mins, then tip onto a board before cutting into wedges.

Coronation hummus

Ingredients

2 x 400g cans chickpeas

1 garlic clove, peeled

5 dried apricots, roughly chopped

2 tsp mild curry powder

1 lemon, zested and juiced

3 tbsp tahini or nut butter of your choice (such as almond, cashew or peanut)

2 tbsp extra virgin olive oil, plus a drizzle

½ small red onion, finely chopped

2 tbsp pomegranate seeds

pinch of nigella seeds

small handful of coriander, mint or parsley leaves

toasted pittas and veg crudités (we used carrots, celery, cucumbers and chicory), to serve

Preparation

STEP 1

Drain the chickpeas over a bowl, reserving the liquid from the can. Tip all but 1 tbsp of the chickpeas into a blender. Add the garlic along with the apricots, curry powder, lemon zest and juice, the tahini or nut butter, oil and some seasoning. Add 4 tbsp of the reserved chickpea liquid and blitz to a smooth paste, adding more liquid if needed. Chill until needed. Will keep chilled for up to two days.

STEP 2

To serve, spoon the hummus onto a plate or into a shallow bowl, using the back of the spoon to create a dip in the middle. Top with the onion, pomegranate seeds, nigella seeds, herbs, reserved 1 tbsp chickpeas and a drizzle of oil. Serve with pittas and crudités for dunking.

Pepper & walnut hummus with veggie dippers

Ingredients

400g can chickpeas, drained

1 garlic clove

1 large roasted red pepper from a jar (not in oil), about 100g

1 tbsp tahini paste

juice ½ lemon

4 walnut halves, chopped

2 courgettes, cut into batons

2 carrots, cut into batons

2 celery sticks, cut into batons

Preparation

STEP 1

Put the chickpeas, garlic, pepper, tahini and lemon juice in a bowl. Blitz with a hand blender or in a food processor to make a thick purée. Stir in the walnuts. Pack into pots, if you like, and serve with the veggie sticks. Will keep in the fridge for two days, although the vegetables are best prepared fresh to preserve their vitamins.

Rosemary, garlic & chilli popcorn

Ingredients

2 tbsp rapeseed oil

2 garlic cloves, lightly bashed

1 tsp chipotle or other chilli flakes

½ small bunch of rosemary, finely chopped

150g popcorn kernels

Preparation

STEP 1

Heat the oil in a saucepan over a medium heat, then fry the garlic, chilli and rosemary for 2-3 mins. Remove from the heat, set aside and leave the oil to infuse for 30 mins.

STEP 2

Cook the popcorn according to pack instructions. Scoop the garlic out of the infused oil and discard. Toss the popcorn with the oil, then season and serve straightaway.

Chickpea Bombay-style mix

Ingredients

60g curried chickpeas (see recipe below)

1 tbsp unsalted peanuts

1 tsp raisins

Preparation

STEP 1

Mix the curried chickpeas (see recipe here) with the unsalted peanuts. Place in the oven at 200C/180C fan/gas 6 for 10 mins, then mix with the raisins.

Tuna Niçoise protein pot

Ingredients

1 large egg

80g green beans

1 tomato, amber or red, quartered

120g can tuna in spring water

1½ -2 tbsp French dressing

Preparation

STEP 1

Boil the egg for 8-10 mins depending on if you want
a soft or hard yolk, then at the same time steam the
green beans for 6 mins above the pan until tender.
Cool the egg and beans under running water then
carefully shell and quarter the egg. Leave to cool.

STEP 2

Tip the beans into a large packed lunch pot. Top with the tomato, tuna and quartered egg and spoon on the French dressing. Seal until ready to eat (see tip below).

Indian oven chips

Ingredients

1kg floury potatoes such as Maris Piper, peeled and cut into chunky chips

½ tsp turmeric

3 tbsp sunflower oil

thumb-sized piece of ginger, peeled and chopped, or finely grated into a paste

3 garlic cloves, peeled and chopped, or finely grated into a paste

1 tsp fennel seeds

generous pinch of cayenne pepper

Preparation

STEP 1

The day before you plan to eat them, tip the potatoes into a pan of cold water and add the turmeric and pinch of salt. Bring to the boil, and simmer gently for 2-3 mins until just cooked. Drain, leave to cool, then chill overnight if you can.

STEP 2

Heat oven to 200C/180C fan/gas 6. Drizzle 1 tbsp of the oil in a shallow roasting tin (preferably non-stick), and place in the oven. Pour the rest of the oil into a large bowl and add the ginger, garlic, fennel seeds and cayenne pepper. Tip the cold chips into the bowl and gently toss with your fingers until evenly coated. Remove the tray from the oven and scatter over the chips. Use a spatula to coat the chips in the hot oil, then lay them out in a single layer and roast for 30 mins. Use the spatula to turn, then return to the oven for 15 mins until crisp and golden.

Hummus snack packs

Ingredients

400g can chickpeas, drained, liquid reserved

1 garlic clove

½ tsp ground cumin

1 tsp ground coriander

1-2 tbsp lemon juice

1 tbsp extra virgin olive oil

2 x 200g bags rainbow carrots or 4 regular carrots

2 x small cucumbers

Preparation

STEP 1

Tip the chickpeas and garlic into a bowl with the cumin, coriander, 1 tbsp lemon juice and the oil. Add 2 tbsp of the reserved liquid from the chickpeas, then blitz using a hand blender until smooth. If the blender is struggling, add another splash of the liquid. Season and add a little more lemon juice if needed.

STEP 2

Spoon the hummus into four small containers. Will keep covered and chilled for up to three days. Slice the carrots and cucumber into batons when you're ready to eat and serve with the hummus.

Pakora

Ingredients

1 green chilli, chopped

thumb-sized piece ginger, roughly chopped

1 tomato, roughly chopped

200g gram flour

1 ½ tsp chilli powder

1 ½ tsp garam masala

1 ½ tsp ground coriander

2 medium potatoes, peeled, halved and thinly sliced, then halved into quarter moons

½ aubergine, thinly sliced, then halved into quarter moons

½ cauliflower, cut into florets

1 large onion, finely sliced

½ lemon, juiced

vegetable oil, for frying

chutney, to serve

Preparation

STEP 1

Heat oven to 120C/100C fan/ gas 1/2. Make a paste by blitzing the chilli, ginger and tomato together, then set aside.

STEP 2

Mix the gram flour with the spices. Add all the prepared vegetables and toss in the mix. Slowly add 150ml water until the batter coats the vegetables – they should be well coated, but not swimming in it.

STEP 3

Add the tomato mixture and get your hands in there, mixing well until everything is incorporated. Add a little lemon juice and seasoning.

STEP 4

Heat the oil to 180C. Take a handful of the mix and squeeze it into a loose little ball, to ensure the vegetables stick to each other when lowered in the oil. Use a spoon to carefully drop the ball into the oil.

STEP 5

Fry for about 4 mins until golden and crispy, then taste to test for seasoning and consistency. You may also need to add a little water or gram our to the mixture at this point if your tester ball didn't hold together. Repeat, frying the remaining mixture in batches.

STEP 6

Drain on kitchen paper and keep warm in the oven as you go. Serve immediately with chutney.

Masala omelette muffins

Ingredients

olive oil, for greasing

2 medium courgettes, coarsely grated

6 large eggs

2 large or 4 small garlic cloves, finely grated

1 red chilli, deseeded and finely chopped

1 tsp chilli powder

1 tsp ground cumin

1 tsp ground coriander

handful fresh coriander, chopped

125g frozen peas

40g feta

Preparation

STEP 1

Heat oven to 220C/200C fan/ gas 7 and lightly oil four 200ml ramekins. Grate the courgettes and squeeze really well, removing as much liquid as possible. Put all the Ingredients except the feta in a large jug and mix really well.

STEP 2

Pour into the ramekins, scatter with the feta and bake on a baking sheet for 20-25 mins until risen and set. You can serve the muffins hot or cold with salad, slaw or cooked vegetables.

Date & peanut butter dip

Ingredients

1 tbsp crunchy peanut butter (30g)

2 dates, finely chopped (10g)

120g bio yogurt

1-2 sticks celery, cut into shorter, thinner lengths

1 green pepper, deseeded and cut into strips

Preparation

STEP 1

Mash the peanut butter and dates together using a fork, then stir in the yogurt. Divide between two small bowls, or pots with lids for packing into lunchboxes. Will keep covered and chilled for up to three days. Serve with the vegetables for dipping.

Chicken skewers with tzatziki

Ingredients

4 skinless chicken breasts

1 lemon

2 tsp oregano

1 garlic clove

1 small yellow pepper

1 small red pepper

wholemeal tortilla wraps, to serve

baby spinach leaves, to serve

few sprigs flat-leaf parsley, to serve

For the tzatziki

½ cucumber

¼ garlic clove

4 tbsp Greek yogurt

1 tbsp extra virgin olive oil

You will need

eight bamboo skewers

Preparation

STEP 1

Soak eight bamboo skewers in water. Using sharp kitchen scissors, chop the chicken into small pieces. Pop into a plastic box with a lid. Pare strips of lemon zest from the lemon using a vegetable peeler, then juice the lemon as well. Add both the peel and the juice to the chicken in the box along with the oregano and the garlic, crushed in. Season generously, mix and put in the fridge for 15 mins with the lid on. Deseed and chop the peppers into similar-sized pieces to those of the chicken.

STEP 2

Heat a griddle pan to high while you get the chicken out. Discard the lemon zest and thread the chicken onto the skewers, alternating every few bits of chicken with a piece of red pepper followed by a piece of yellow pepper. Griddle for 10 mins, turning halfway.

STEP 3

While the skewers are cooking, make the tzatziki. Get a box grater and a bowl. Cut the cucumber into long lengths, discarding the watery seedy core. Grate into the bowl, then grate the ¼ garlic clove. Season generously and stir in the Greek yogurt. Drizzle with a little extra virgin olive oil.

STEP 4

Serve the skewers hot off the griddle with the dip, or take the chicken and peppers off the skewers, leave to cool and pack into wholemeal wraps spread with a little tzatziki and rolled up with baby spinach and a few picked leaves of parsley.

Air fryer chicken wings

Ingredients

1kg chicken wings

1 tbsp sunflower or olive oil

seasoning of your choice (use salt and pepper, or ½-1 tsp of either smoky BBQ, ras-el-hanout, garlic granules, celery salt or garam masala)

dipping sauce, to serve (optional)

Preparation

STEP 1

Separate each chicken wing in two at the joint, removing the wing tips if you like using sharp kitchen scissors. Toss the chicken wings in the oil and seasoning, then tip into an air fryer (you can either use one with a paddle, or arrange them on the tray of your air fryer if it doesn't have a paddle).

STEP 2

Program the air fryer to cook for 35 mins. Check the wings are tender and cooked through – they should be almost falling off the bone – and cook for a further 5 mins if needed. The skin should have bubbled and crisped up, and any excess fat from the chicken will have dripped off into base of the fryer (discard this). Don't leave the chicken in the fryer, or the steam will make the skin soft again.

Immediately tip into a bowl and serve with sauce for dipping.

Cauliflower & squash fritters with mint & feta dip

Ingredients

100g gram (chickpea) flour

1 tsp turmeric

1 tsp ground cumin

small bunch coriander, finely chopped (optional)

oil, for shallow frying

150g natural yogurt

1 garlic clove, crushed

75g vegetarian feta, mashed

2 tbsp finely chopped mint

pitta breads and salad, to serve

For the roast cauliflower & squash base

1 cauliflower, split into florets, the stalk cut into cubes

½ large butternut squash, cut into cubes

1 tbsp oil

Preparation

STEP 1

Heat oven to 180C/160C fan/gas 4. Toss the cauliflower and squash in oil and spread it out on a large oven tray. Roast for 25 mins, or until tender. If you're making the base ahead of time, you can leave it to cool at this stage then freeze in an airtight container for up to a month. (Defrost fully before using in the next step.)

STEP 2

Put the flour in a bowl and gradually stir in 125-150ml water to make a batter as thick as double cream. Stir in the turmeric and cumin and some seasoning. Break up the cauliflower and squash a little and mix it gently into the batter. Add the coriander, if using.

STEP 3

Heat a little oil in a frying pan and when it is hot, drop 2 heaped tbsps of the mixture into the pan, spaced apart. Fry until the fritters are dark golden, about 2-3 mins each side. Remove, keep warm and repeat with the remaining batter.

STEP 4

Mix the yogurt with the garlic, feta and mint. Serve the fritters with the mint & feta dip, some salad and pitta breads.

Healthy egg & chips

Ingredients

500g potatoes, diced

2 shallots, sliced

1 tbsp olive oil

2 tsp dried crushed oregano or 1 tsp fresh leaves

200g small mushroom

4 eggs

Preparation

STEP 1

Heat oven to 200C/fan 180C/gas 6. Tip the potatoes and shallots into a large, non-stick roasting tin, drizzle with the oil, sprinkle over the oregano, then mix everything together well. Bake for 40-45 mins (or until starting to go brown), add the mushrooms, then cook for a further 10 mins until the potatoes are browned and tender.

STEP 2

Make four gaps in the vegetables and crack an egg into each space. Return to the oven for 3-4 mins or until the eggs are cooked to your liking.

JUST ONE FINAL THING TO ADDRESS BEFORE YOU GO!

In conclusion, it's evident that diet plays a crucial role in managing Postural Orthostatic Tachycardia Syndrome (POTS). By adopting a balanced diet rich in fluids, electrolytes, and nutrients, individuals with POTS can potentially alleviate symptoms and enhance their quality of life. However, it's essential to tailor dietary changes to individual needs and consult with healthcare professionals for personalized recommendations. Further research into the specific effects of different dietary components on POTS symptoms could provide valuable insights for optimizing treatment strategies in the future.

www.ingramcontent.com/pod-product-compliance
Lightning Source LLC
Chambersburg PA
CBHW061040250726
48653CB00001B/183